Makeup Tutorial

A Manual On All The Secrets Artistry And Application Of Makeup

By SARAH HOMES

ISBN: 9798534276077

DEDICATION

To Annie Klose.

CONTENTS

ACKNOWLEDGMENTS

Thank you
Lekky Design and Beauty.

CHAPTER ONE
INTRODUCTION

In this volume, I will be showing you how to do a full face makeup. I will show you exactly what you need to complete a beautiful face makeup. I will show you the set of brushes to try and some blenders and products to experiment with. I will give tips and techniques on how to achieve an amazing finish. We are going to start with eyeshadow, and then, we do the rest of the face.

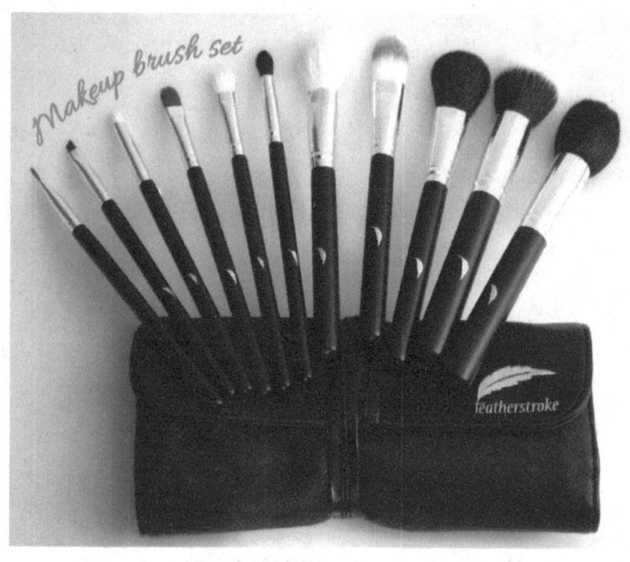
Makeup brush set
featherstroke

CHAPTER TWO
COMPLETE EYE MAKEUP

We are going to do the eyeshadow first, before we do the face as I said. We will start with the brows. I want you to know one thing about working on the brows. I found the best starting point long before now and that is lining the upper side before the lower. That's the recommended starting point.

There is another thing you need to observe even before you start your lining. That is the condition of your skin. If the skin is the oily type, you need to dry off the oil in that area first before ever you start lining it. This is very essential, especially if you are using eye pencil for lining.

To dry the oil you can do one of these two things. 1. Put some powder on the brow area to dry it. Make sure the brow area is very dry. And 2. As an alternative, wash the face with soap and dry thoroughly with a towel and make sure the area is also very, very dry. Then, you can start lining.

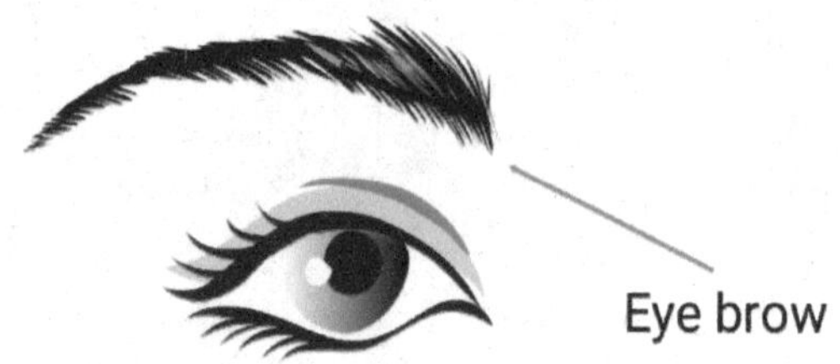

Keep in mind that we want everything to appear very natural. So, if your brows are wide around the inner corner, shave off the sharp edge of the upper side of the brows. If your brow is curved at the top of that inner corner, you don't need to shave. And when you are lining, leave a small space around the inner corner. This ensures that you have a more natural curve around the inner corner instead of a block shape.

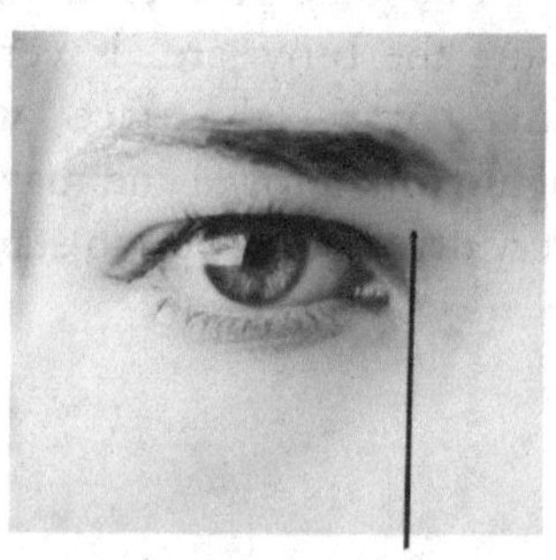

Inner corner

After shaving off, that is if you have that wide hair on your brows, and after leaving that small bit of space, then keep lining until it's perfect. Then you apply a primer. Here are some top picks for you: Tatcha The Silk, The Ordinary, e.l.f, Glossier, Fenty Beauty and Benefit.

But there is something important about the primer you chose to use. I don't recommend that you use a shining primer. No. A matte primer gives the best results. This is a technique that gives an amazing natural finish, that feather-like beauty. That's the result.

Apart from primer, you can also use hair glue or soap to prime your brow, if that is what you prefer.

Next, begin to brush through the brow. Use the set of brow hair brush to brush through.

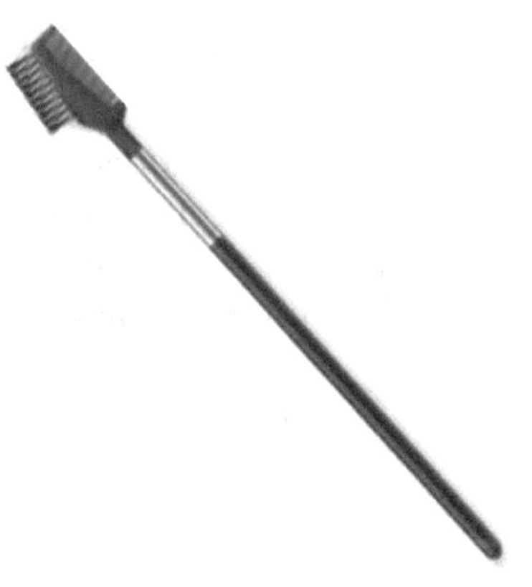

That is it. After you have applied primer, this

is what you do. Keep brushing through the eyebrows using this brush. Your brow becomes more visible. Keep brushing through. The brushing separates the hair as you brush through. Especially if you have a bushy brow, the hair becomes more like feathers and quite awesome.

When you have finished brushing, gently press it so that the brows stay that way until it dries or set.

Now, the primer is dry. You want to start filling. Remember that our goal is to have a very natural finish. So, don't let the brows be too dark. Fill in only the area where you think there are spaces.

After filling in the spaces, next is aligning the brows. Yes, we need to balance them. Here we are going to use concealer. There are also different makes of concealer. Here are also some examples. Nars Radiant, Tarte Shape, L. A. Girl, NYX, Maybelline and Almay Clear.

It is best to use a concealer shade that is about two levels lighter than your own skin tone.

And don't use a fluffy brush for this. Even if you pinch a fluffy brush together, you can never get the result you want. Use a quite angled brush instead. That's best for cleaning or concealing to give you the perfect shape.

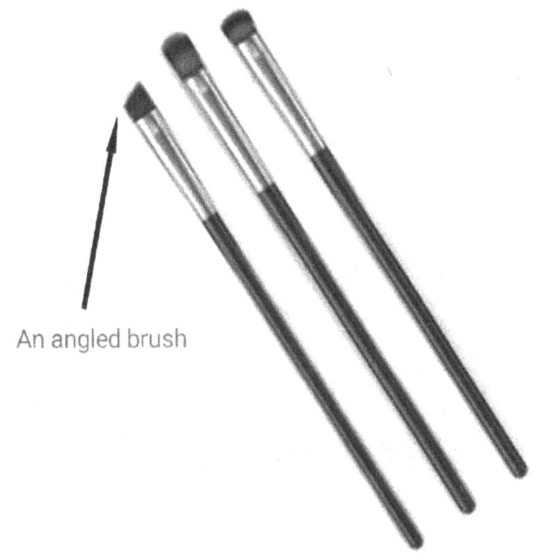

An angled brush

To conceal the upper part of the brows, some make up artists favor using foundation instead of a concealer. And I found this to work best, myself. You know, later on, you are going to blend. Especially for beginners, it will be easier to blend foundation at the upper side than to blend concealer. So, use foundation to align the upper side.

Next set the eyelids. Use the same concealer you just used for cleaning and aligning your brows to set the eyelids itself. Then blend in thoroughly. This prep is important before you start applying the eyeshadow.

Let's now apply eyeshadow. Open and see the colors of your transition. You see dark, chocolate, orange and other lighter colors. Apart from the colors, there is something I want to call your attention to. You can see that some of the transitions are shimmery, that is shining. Others are more stable sensation or are matte. That is what I want to show you.

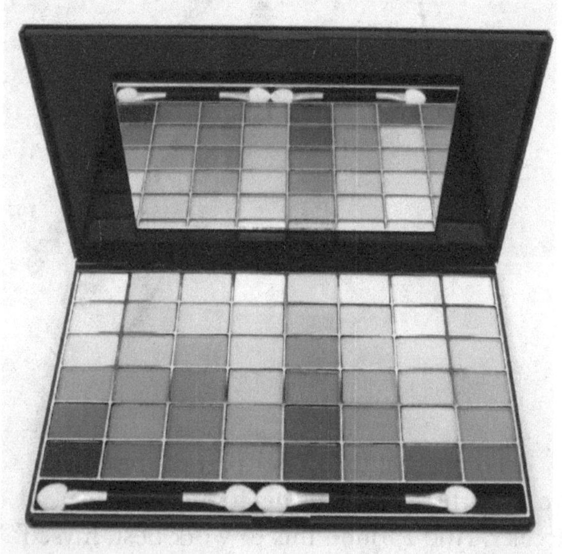

Never should you start your shading with that glossy or shimmery transition. Always, at any time, start transitioning with matte shades.

Remember too, I said before that you should make sure you blend your eyelids very smoothly when setting it. This ensure that there are no creases when you put the eyeshadow shades. And the best brush to use for blending your transition shades must be a round fluffy brush. But where do you start putting the transition?

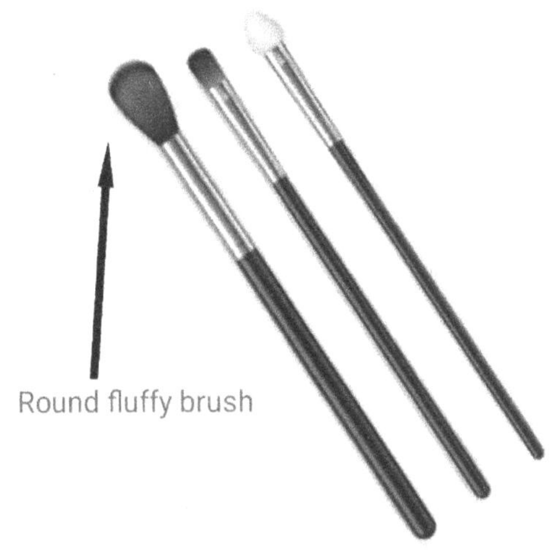

Don't start from the inner corner. No. Start from the outer corner. From the outer side, you keep going inside. You keep moving towards the inner corner.

So, let's start. Remember, from the outer corner. Pick a dark color, but not black. As a beginner, don't start with black. Pick something chocolatey shade to start. And from the outer corner.

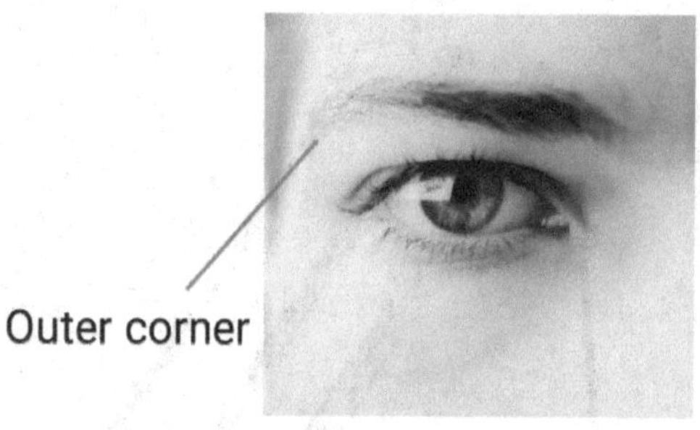

Before we continue to apply the eyeshadow, I want you to know something. As you continue to practice, you can begin to adjust your starting colors from chocolate to more darker shades. In days to come in the future, you will be able to start with black and it won't give you any problem. But as a beginner, start your transitioning with a chocolate shade.

So, let's continue. Settle that chocolate shade on the outer corner. Then, pick another shade that's a little bit lighter than the chocolate, a more subtle brown or so. Apply it a little inside following the first darker shade we began with as our first transition. And then, blend them in smoothly. Blend the two in thoroughly. Ensure there are no hash lines.

Next pick another color. This should be lighter than the last one you used, maybe orange or so. Put it next to the last one we did. Blend again. Blend it smoothly again.

So, that is how it goes. To summarize this step, start with a darker color at the outer corner. Then, move towards the inner corner with shades that have very subtle difference. The shades get brighter as you approach the inner corner. Blend as you go. Ensure to blend very smoothly, no hash lines. You can use the same brush you used to clean the brows with concealer earlier. It doesn't matter. It even helps to maintain the same color. But when you want to blend the edges, a smaller fluffy brush is better. Blend smoothly. With little force, blend, turning the brush round and round. Yes, with very small force.

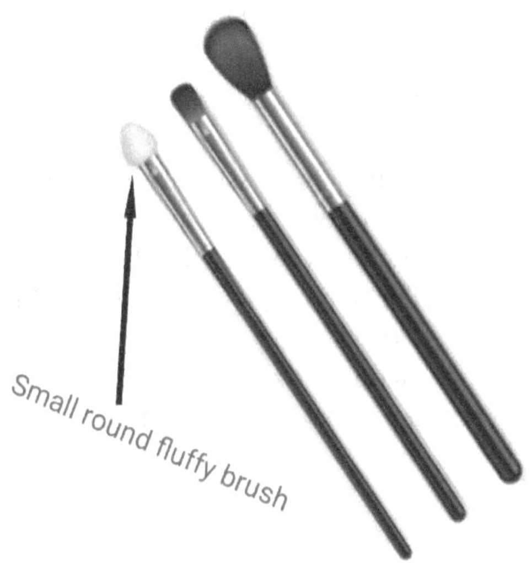

When you are done blending, apply eyeliner again. Apply up the brows until it meets the very first shade of transition. Then, blend the eyeliner in with the first transitioning shade. Or you can draw the eyeliner longer down, if you prefer. This will require some artistic skills to determine what longer winger is ok for your face. Is it a straight line or an arch? If you get the right one for your face, it will be awesome. Then, blend it in with a small angle brush to the first transition shade too. You may also decide not to extend the line. If you do not extend the line, then blend in the eyeliner with a smaller round fluffy brush.

It's now time to put the falsies. Now, something comes before putting the falsies. That's a thickener for the eyelashes. Use Mascara, use what is enough to hold the falsies. This is because you don't want to put more mascara after you fix the falsies. If mascara touches the falsies, trust me, you are not going to like the shape.

Also, many professional makeup artists, advise that you shift your falsies away a little from the inner corner. That will make the finishing natural. And it's true. The technique is amazing. But if the falsies are too close to the inner corner, you see, it becomes quite awful. Set the failsies to the thickened eyelashes and then press it against it to make sure they align perfectly.

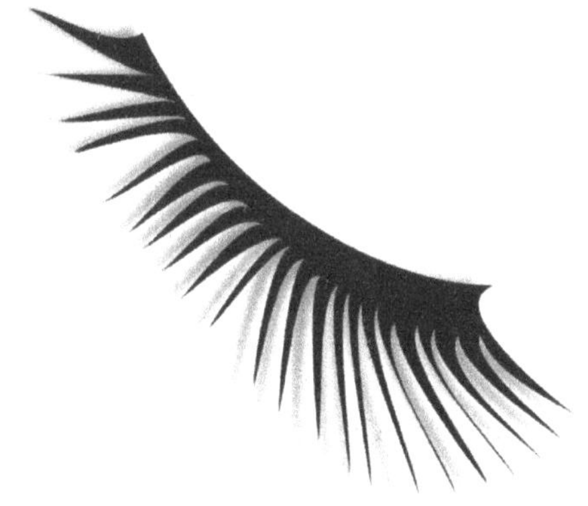

That is how we finish our eyeshadow. We are now going to move over to the rest of the face.

CHAPTER THREE
FACE MAKEUP

FACE MAKEUP

What should we consider at the beginning before starting to do the face? Well, you need to realize that all skin textures are not the same. Some of us have dry skins while others are damp or oily. We need to prepare the skin first. For this, we use moisturizer. But for those with more oil on the skin, they need to wash the skin and then dry very well before applying primer.

Here are some examples of moisturizer makes you can use. Vaseline Advanced Repair, Olay, No7, Cetaphil, Vanicream.

I'm sure you have a good sunscreen. If not buy one before you apply moisturizer. Cetaphil and Vanicream are also good for sun screening for sensitive skin. EltaMD and Aveeno are other good sunscreens.

And hoping you have a moisturizer of your choice, rub some on your face and massage. Massage it thoroughly into your skin. Let it set after you massage. Always remember to do this step.

Next is Application of primer. Once you selected your preferred seller, massage the primer in first. But some experts say that primer should not be massaged with the same intensity as you did the moisturizer. They say rub lightly and just leave it like that. But I massage very well and get good results too. But you can experiment with the two. It's always good to try something new.

Some people with deep smile lines may have problem blending that area of the face. If you realize that, put more primer there at the smile lines and tap it in very well. Make sure they are filled out thoroughly. When the primer is set, you can then apply foundation over it.

Here are some of the blenders you can use to put foundation. Beautyblender, e.l.f. Total Face, Wet n Wild, Beauty Bakeries. Make sure they are quite soft. Wet the blender with water. But don't let it be dripping. Remove excess water by squeezing it.

For foundation, you can select from these options. Giorgio Armani, CoverGirl and Olay Simply Ageless, No7, It, Laura Mercier, Maybelline New York.

Once you have your preferred foundation, apply it to you face. Use your already damped blender to, just be tapping to blend. Just a tap for an area. Just a tap for one side. Keep tapping. Don't use too much. That won't give you a good result. You will have problem blending quite smoothly. Using small product is always the best thing to do. Always very small amount of product. Keep tapping until it blends in. Include the neck. Tap on it, blend it in with the face to get your neck a uniform tone with the face. Your forehead should not be neglected too. But use even much smaller amount on your forehead, as small as you can. Blend in everything, so you don't have separate skin tones for your head, neck and face.

After blending in the foundation, what you do next is emphasize some areas of your face. Use a concealer for the highlight. Use the one you used earlier to align your brows. As usual, very small product for highlight.

Immediately blend each place that you highlighted. Don't wait until you apply concealer on all the places you want to highlight before you blend. Apply, blend. Apply, blend. Apply under your eyes, on the bridge of your nose, your forehead. Don't allow it to dry while you are blending in. This method works well for you.

After Blending in the highlight that we did with our concealer, use setting powder to set the places that we highlighted. Here are some examples of setting powder names. Danessa Myricks, Beauty Bakeries, Laura Mercier, Ilia Soft, and Milk.

Just dip your soft blender into the setting powder. Blow out any access, that is excess powder first before you begin to use this setting powder that is remaining on the soft blender. Blend by pressing in all the areas. Just like that. You will finally have a perfect finish.

So, always set all the areas you highlighted. You remember, those were under your eyes, your forehead, the bridge of your nose or the middle of your upper lip. These were the places you highlighted with the concealer and also blended in. Set all of them with the setting powder.

It is when you have done the setting of those highlights before you can start sculpting.

Sculpting actually involves giving shape to your face. Here are some product makes you can use for contour. E.l.f, L'Oréal Paris, Aj Crimson, Fenty Beauty. This should be up to 2 levels darker than your skin tone to make a difference. Apply a very small force to contour. And use a fluffy brush to sculpt your cheeks and your forehead. And be sure to blend in the contours. For the nose, put the contour shade on the tip of your nose only. It shouldn't be all over the bridge of your nose, just the tip of your nose.

The contouring continue. Put a visible highlight on the nose. But it should be around the tip. Then, use a small angled brush to reverse the line. We don't need a shouting light. At the same time, we need one not too obvious to sculpt the nose. That is why we want to reverse the contour. Expert beauticians just found this out and it's very amazing. Use the setting powder we are applying. Put on the two sides of your nose. And remember, with very little force. And you can use your finger to blend that in.

If you use this technique, you won't have any harsh line around your nose after you sculpt.

It is now time to decide the size you need your nose to look in the eyes of whoever sees you after. If you want it to be thin, you can sculpt and have the nose look thin. If you want to look to have a bigger nose, your sculpting will also determine that by making the line wider a little bit. When you have reversed the contour of your nose, highlight the bridge of the nose next. Use a smaller fluffy brush and the same setting powder and choose your preferred size. And blend the sides of your nose until you have a flawless finish.

Now, you need to set the entire face. The product to use here is the face setting spray. If you have your preferred one, spray it on your face. Keep turning your face. Let it go round your entire face.

After the setting spray, highlight again. Highlight the bridge of your nose, the peak of your cheeks and the center of your upper lip. Next, use your finger to blend it in smoothly. That keeps it from being that sharp or very obvious. Let's dive to the lips now.

Now, if your lower lip is thinner than the upper lip, start your lining with the upper lip. And if it's otherwise, the reverse should be the case. It works better that way. Remember the liner we used for the brows earlier? That's going to be perfect for lining the lips. But if the lining is not as vivid as you desire, pick a pigment from your eyebrows shades that matches the color of your lining and it shouldn't be a glossy or shimmery shade.

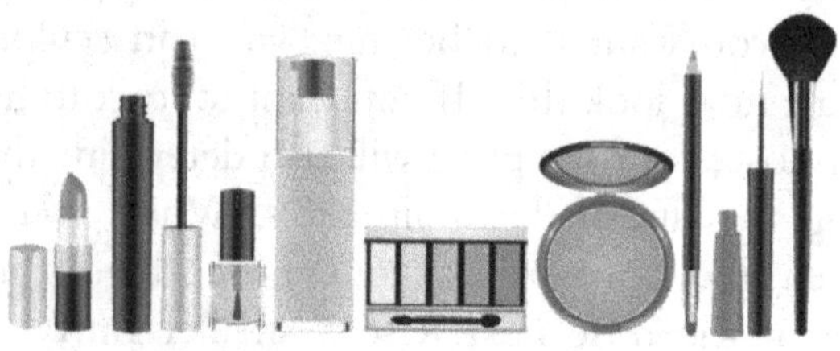

Start with the lower lip accordingly. And to balance the lip sizes, enlarge the lining of the thinner lip by overlaying the initial line until you can look and feel they are balanced.

Finally, you do the lips after the lining. Use a quality lipstick, concentrating on the bigger lip. Then, smear it to the other lip by stamping the lips and disengaging them, slowly, or you just smudge, and then blend with a finger. If you want the lip to pop, put a small amount of golden shade after you smudged. After adding the gold, blend in very well with your finger. It will give you that awesome pop you want.

CHAPTER FOUR
CONCLUSION

So, this is all we have for a full face makeup tutorial at this time. I tried to be very detailed. I showed you all the techniques, the exact tips and tricks to help you do it right. I also showed you the tools and the products you need. You can now go ahead and try what you learned. Hopefully, you will come out with that amazing result that you desire.

APPRECIATION

Thank you for reading our book. We appreciate you
– **Sarah Homes,** Author.

If it's pleases you, can you please, give us a minute or two of your time to share how you feel about this tutorial? We will be very grateful if you are able to represent this by star rating also. Thanks once again